Happy Marriage

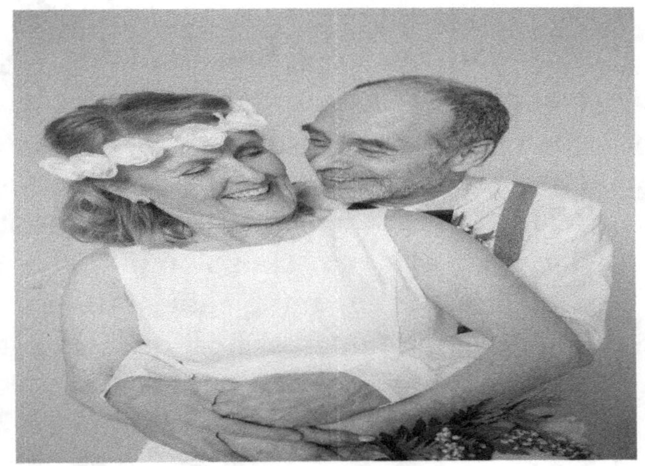

A Guide on Principles of a Joyful and Everlasting Marriage

Marissa Erickson

TABLE OF CONTENTS

Happy Marriage 1

A Guide on Principles of a Joyful and
Everlasting Marriage 1

Copyright page 2

INTRODUCTION 5

Chapter 1 11

Building Open and Honest Communication 11

Chapter 2 17

Nurturing Trust and Mutual Respect 17

"Nurturing Trust and Mutual Respect" is a fundamental principle that forms the foundation of a happy and successful marriage. Trust is the cornerstone of any healthy relationship, as it involves having confidence in your partner's honesty, reliability, and intentions. In a marriage, trust is built over time through open communication, transparency, and consistently keeping promises. 17

Chapter 3 23

Embracing Growth and Change Together 23

Chapter 4 29

Cultivating Shared Goals and Values 29

Chapter 5 33

Fostering Intimacy and Romance 33

Chapter 6 41

Resolving Conflict with Grace 41

Chapter 7 47

Forgiveness and Compromise 47

These two aspects contribute significantly to

the longevity and strength of a marital relationship. Let's delve into each concept in more detail: **47**

Forgiveness: 47

Compromise   50

Chapter 8   **59**

Prioritizing Self-Care and Individuality   59

Prioritizing self-care and individuality within a marriage is crucial for maintaining a healthy and fulfilling relationship. While the idea of focusing on oneself might seem counterintuitive to a partnership, it's actually a key element in ensuring both partners remain content and capable of contributing positively to the relationship.   **59**

Chapter 9   **65**

Embracing Laughter and Playfulness   65

Chapter 10   **73**

Sustaining Marriage Commitment   73

Chapter 11   **79**

Faithfulness   79

Chapter 12   **87**

LOVE   87

Conclusion   **95**

INTRODUCTION

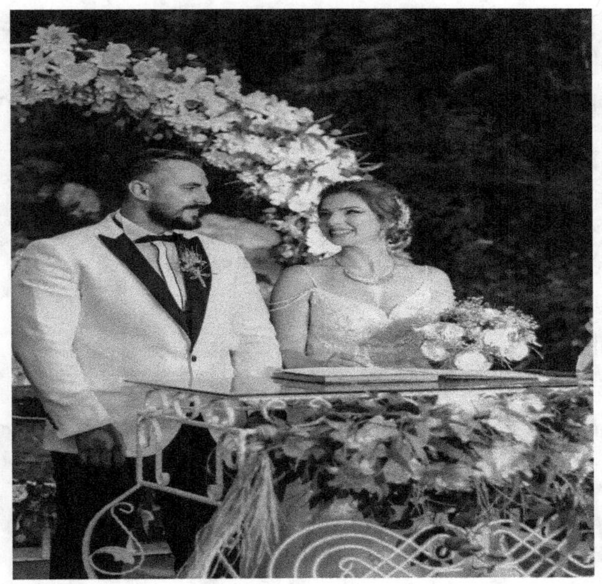

In a world of constant change, the pursuit of a happy and everlasting marriage remains a timeless aspiration. "Happy Marriage" delves into the guiding principles that form the foundation of a strong, loving, and enduring marital relationship. Through the exploration of communication, trust, commitment, and growth, this book offers insights to help couples navigate the beautiful journey of marriage.

A happy marriage is a timeless union of two individuals who embark on a journey together, not merely as partners in life but as soulmates, companions, and confidants. It is a sacred bond built upon a foundation of love, trust, and mutual respect, enduring the tests of time and trials of life. In a happy marriage, each day is a testament to the power of commitment, where two hearts beat in harmony, sharing dreams, joys, and sorrows, while supporting and uplifting one another. It is a partnership that thrives on open communication, understanding, and compromise, fostering an environment where both partners can grow individually while simultaneously nurturing the growth of their shared love. A happy marriage is not exempt from challenges, but it is defined by the strength and resilience to overcome them, emerging even stronger, bound by an unbreakable connection.

A happy marriage is a union characterized by profound love, unwavering commitment, and a shared journey through life's joys and challenges. It is a testament to the remarkable bond between two individuals who have chosen to embark on this lifelong adventure together, hand in hand. In a world where the dynamics of relationships continually evolve, a truly happy marriage remains a timeless and cherished institution.

At its core, a happy marriage is built upon a foundation of trust and communication. It is the space where both partners can express themselves openly and honestly, knowing that their thoughts and feelings will be heard and respected. In such a marriage, conflicts are seen as opportunities for growth and understanding, rather than as threats to the relationship.

Mutual respect is another essential pillar of a happy marriage. Each partner values the other's uniqueness, appreciating their strengths and accepting their imperfections. This respect extends to the shared goals and dreams that define the couple's journey together. A happy

marriage thrives when both individuals actively
support each other's aspirations and work
together to achieve them.

Laughter and shared moments of joy are the
glue that binds a happy marriage. It's the ability
to find humor even in challenging times, and
the simple pleasures of being together, that
keep the relationship vibrant. This shared
sense of happiness is a testament to the strong
emotional connection between partners.

Moreover, a happy marriage is a partnership
where both individuals contribute to the
well-being of the family unit. It is the
recognition that responsibilities are shared, and
both partners play a crucial role in creating a
harmonious and nurturing environment for
themselves and any potential children.

In addition, a happy marriage is a harmonious blend of love, trust, respect, shared happiness, and mutual support. It's a journey that continually evolves, deepens, and enriches the lives of those who embark on it. When nurtured with care and dedication, a happy marriage becomes a source of enduring joy and fulfillment, demonstrating the incredible power of love in human relationships.

In the intricate tapestry of love and companionship, the principles of a happy marriage are woven with threads of understanding, communication, and unwavering support. As we embark on a journey through these pages, we'll explore how mutual respect, shared goals, and a commitment to growth form the foundation of a resilient and blissful marital union.

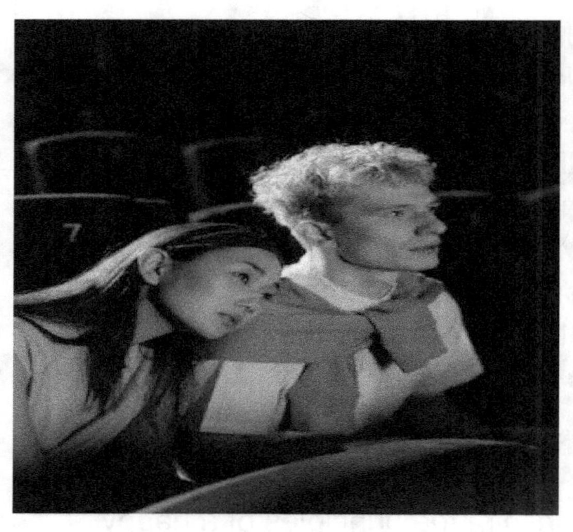

Chapter 1

Building Open and Honest Communication

Every successful marriage is built on strong communication. This chapter explores active listening, expressing emotions, and practicing empathy to foster understanding between partners. Through transparent conversations, couples can create a safe space for each other's thoughts, fears, and dreams, strengthening their connection.

Communication is a cornerstone of a happy marriage. It involves not just talking, but actively listening and understanding each other's thoughts, feelings, and needs. Open and honest communication fosters trust, resolves conflicts, and helps partners grow together. Sharing both joys and challenges allows couples to maintain emotional intimacy and strengthen their connection over time. Effective communication also helps prevent misunderstandings and ensures that both partners feel heard and valued in the relationship.

Building open and honest communication in marriage is essential for a strong and lasting relationship. It involves:

Active Listening: Pay attention to your partner's words, thoughts, and feelings without interrupting. Show empathy and validate their emotions.

Express Yourself: Share your thoughts, feelings, and concerns openly, but do so respectfully. Be clear and direct, avoiding passive-aggressive behavior.

Create a Safe Space: Foster an environment where both partners feel safe to share their true selves without fear of judgment or criticism.

Avoid Assumptions: Instead of assuming, ask for clarification. Misunderstandings often arise from assumptions that aren't accurate.

Nonverbal Communication: Study the facial expressions and body language of others. They frequently express feelings that words might be unable to.

Regular Check-Ins: Set aside time to talk regularly about how you both are feeling and how the relationship is progressing.

Conflict Resolution: Address conflicts calmly and constructively. Instead of placing blame , focus on finding solutions.

Be Patient: Communication takes time and practice. Don't expect perfect communication overnight.

Be Mindful of Tone: The way you say something matters as much as what you say. Avoid a confrontational or accusatory tone.

Celebrate Achievements: Acknowledge and celebrate when you successfully communicate, solve a problem, or reach a compromise.

Remember, building open and honest communication is an ongoing effort. It requires mutual respect, understanding, and a willingness to continuously work on improving the way you interact with each other.

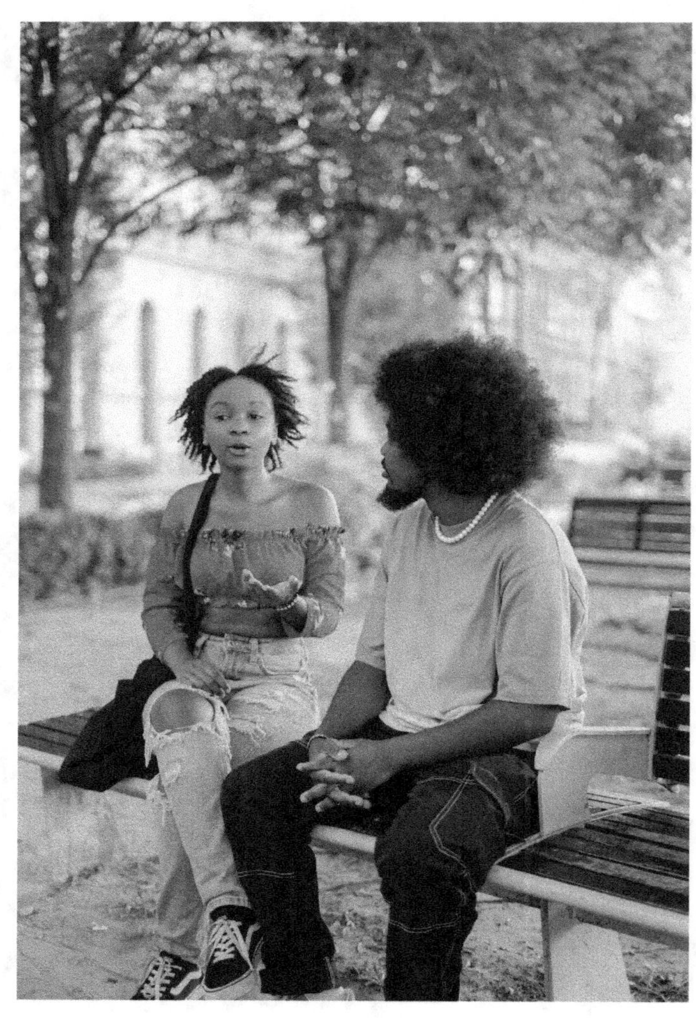

Chapter 2

Nurturing Trust and Mutual Respect

Trust is the bedrock of a lasting marriage. This chapter delves into the significance of trust and respect in a partnership. By maintaining honesty, honoring commitments, and supporting each other's individuality, couples can cultivate a deep sense of trust that binds them together through challenges and triumphs.

"Nurturing Trust and Mutual Respect" is a fundamental principle that forms the foundation of a happy and successful marriage. Trust is the cornerstone of any healthy relationship, as it involves having confidence in your partner's honesty, reliability, and intentions. In a marriage, trust is built over time through open communication, transparency, and consistently keeping promises.

Mutual respect goes hand in hand with trust. It involves valuing your partner's opinions, feelings, and boundaries. Respecting each other's individuality and autonomy is essential, as it ensures that both partners feel valued and acknowledged. When there is mutual respect, disagreements are handled with empathy and sensitivity, avoiding demeaning or hurtful behavior.

To nurture trust and mutual respect in a marriage, it's crucial to:

1. **Communicate openly:** Honest and open communication creates an atmosphere of transparency, making it

easier to discuss any concerns or issues. Sharing thoughts, feelings, and experiences helps partners understand each other better.

2. **Be reliable**: Keeping your promises and commitments demonstrates dependability, reinforcing trust. This applies to both small promises and larger life commitments.

3. **Honor boundaries**: Respecting each other's personal space, opinions, and boundaries shows that you value your partner's individuality. This contributes to a sense of safety within the relationship.

4. **Show appreciation:** Expressing gratitude and acknowledging each other's contributions fosters a sense of worth and respect. Small gestures of

appreciation can go a long way in
maintaining a positive atmosphere.

5. **Empathize and validate:**
Understanding and acknowledging your
partner's emotions, even if you don't
agree, helps build empathy and
demonstrates respect for their feelings.

6. **Resolve conflicts constructively:**
Disagreements are natural in any
relationship. Handling conflicts calmly
and respectfully, while focusing on
finding solutions rather than assigning
blame, strengthens the bond between
partners.

7. **Spend quality time together:** Quality
time builds emotional connection.
Engaging in shared activities and
meaningful conversations deepens your
understanding of each other.

8. **Prioritize each other:** Showing that your partner is a priority in your life reinforces the idea that they are respected and valued.

By consistently practicing these principles, a couple can create an environment of **trust and mutual respect** that fosters a **strong, happy, and lasting marriage.**

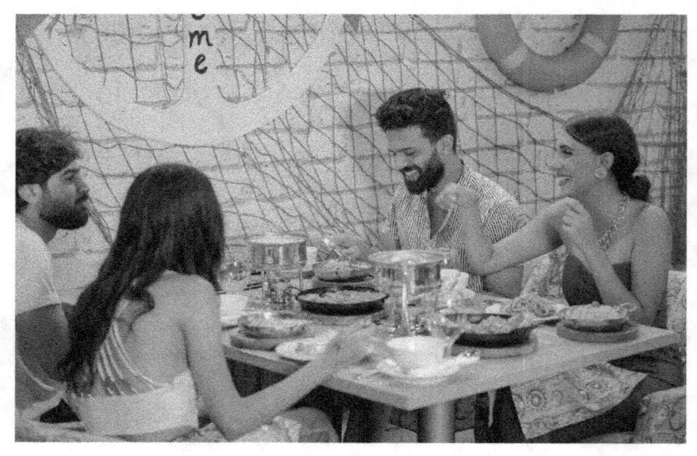

Chapter 3

Embracing Growth and Change Together

Change is inevitable, both within individuals and within a relationship. This chapter discusses the importance of embracing personal and relational growth. Couples are encouraged to evolve alongside each other, celebrating accomplishments and adapting to life's transitions with unwavering support.

"Embracing Growth and Change Together" is a fundamental principle of a happy marriage that recognizes the dynamic nature of both individuals and relationships. It involves a shared commitment to support each other's personal growth, adapt to life's changes, and evolve together as a couple.

In practical terms, this principle involves
several key aspects:

1. **Open Communication:** Couples who
    embrace growth and change
    communicate openly and honestly about
    their aspirations, fears, and evolving
    needs. This fosters an environment of
    trust and understanding, allowing each
    partner to share their desires for
    personal development and changes
    within the relationship.

2. **Supporting Individual** Growth: Healthy
    marriages encourage each partner to
    pursue their individual interests,
    passions, and goals. Partners cheer
    each other on, offering emotional
    support and practical assistance as

needed. This not only enriches the individuals but also strengthens the bond between them.

3. **Flexibility and Adaptability:** Life is full of changes, and a successful marriage acknowledges this reality. Embracing growth and change means being flexible and adaptable in the face of challenges, new circumstances, and unexpected events. Couples who can navigate change together tend to emerge stronger.

4. **Shared Goals and Values:** While embracing growth and change as individuals, couples also need to establish shared goals and values. This provides a sense of direction and purpose, helping them navigate

changes in alignment with their
collective vision for the future.

5. **Learning and Self-Reflection:** Partners
committed to growth actively seek
opportunities to learn and improve
themselves. This includes being open to
feedback, engaging in self-reflection,
and recognizing areas where personal
development is possible.

6. **Empathy and Patience:** Embracing
change often requires empathy and
patience. Partners may go through
different phases of transformation, and
understanding each other's journeys
with empathy and offering patience can
smooth the process.

7. **Embracing Challenges as
Opportunities:** Challenges and
conflicts are inevitable in any marriage.

Couples who embrace growth and change see these challenges as opportunities for growth and learning, rather than as obstacles to their happiness.

8. **Renewing the Relationship:** Over time, couples change, and so do their relationships. Embracing growth means periodically reassessing and renewing the relationship dynamics, keeping it fresh and aligned with the current needs and aspirations of both partners.

Ultimately, **"Embracing Growth and Change Together"** is about recognizing that a successful marriage is a journey of mutual evolution. It requires a commitment to support each other's individual growth while navigating life's twists and turns as a united team.

Chapter 4

Cultivating Shared Goals and Values

Shared goals and values provide a roadmap for a harmonious partnership. This chapter emphasizes the significance of aligning ambitions and values, which helps couples navigate decisions and challenges while maintaining a sense of unity and purpose.

Certainly! Cultivating shared goals and values in a marriage is about building a strong foundation of mutual understanding, cooperation, and harmony. Here's a more detailed explanation of this principle:

1. **Alignment of Aspirations:** When partners in a marriage share common goals, they create a sense of unity and purpose. These goals can encompass various aspects of life, such as career

ambitions, family planning, financial stability, and personal growth. By discussing and setting these goals together, couples can work collaboratively towards achieving them, providing a sense of accomplishment and mutual support along the way.

2. **Strengthened Communication:** Engaging in conversations about shared goals and values requires open and honest communication. This practice encourages both partners to listen actively and express themselves clearly. This, in turn, enhances their overall communication skills and deepens their connection. Regular discussions about their individual aspirations and how they fit into their joint vision allow them to better understand each other's perspectives.

3. **Conflict Resolution:** Disagreements and conflicts are inevitable in any relationship. However, when couples share common goals and values, these differences can be resolved more effectively. Having a shared purpose helps them approach conflicts with a mindset of finding solutions that align

with their collective vision. They can focus on the bigger picture rather than getting bogged down in trivial disagreements.

4. **Mutual Growth:** Shared goals and values encourage couples to support each other's personal development. When both partners are committed to each other's growth and success, they create an environment of encouragement and empowerment. This can lead to both individuals becoming their best selves, both independently and as a couple.

5. **Emotional Connection:** A sense of shared purpose fosters a deeper emotional connection. Couples who work towards common objectives feel a strong sense of companionship and intimacy. This shared journey can create lasting memories and strengthen the emotional bond between partners.

6. **Building Trust and Respect:** When couples have shared goals and values, it demonstrates a level of trust and respect for each other's opinions and aspirations. This foundation of trust

forms the basis for a resilient and enduring relationship.

7. **Long-Term Stability:** Cultivating shared goals and values contributes to the long-term stability of the marriage. As life evolves and circumstances change, having a common direction helps the couple adapt and navigate challenges together. This reduces the likelihood of drifting apart due to differing priorities.

In essence, cultivating shared goals and values is about creating a roadmap for the marriage, a roadmap that both partners are excited about and committed to following. It's not just about having similar interests, but also about aligning core values, beliefs, and life aspirations. This principle helps couples build a strong, fulfilling, and happy partnership that can weather the ups and downs of life.

Chapter 5

Fostering Intimacy and Romance

Intimacy goes beyond physical connection—it encompasses emotional closeness, vulnerability, and romance. This chapter explores ways to keep the flame of passion alive, from simple gestures of affection to nurturing a deep emotional connection that strengthens over time.

Fostering intimacy and romance is a crucial principle for a happy marriage. Intimacy involves emotional closeness, vulnerability, and sharing of thoughts and feelings. Romance adds excitement, affection, and a sense of passion to the relationship. These elements help maintain a strong bond and create a deeper connection between partners.

Cultivating intimacy requires effective communication, active listening, and empathy. Sharing life's ups and downs, discussing dreams and fears, and showing genuine interest in each other's lives contribute to emotional intimacy. This kind of connection helps partners understand each other better, build trust, and feel supported.

Romance injects vitality into the marriage. Simple gestures like surprise date nights, handwritten notes, or small gifts can rekindle the spark. Regular quality time together and maintaining physical affection, even through touch and cuddling, help sustain the romantic aspect of the relationship.

It's important to adapt to changing circumstances. As life evolves, so do relationship dynamics. Nurturing intimacy and romance might require creativity to accommodate busy schedules, work-related stress, or the presence of children. Finding shared hobbies, going on adventures, or prioritizing alone time can help keep the romance alive.

Ultimately, the combination of emotional intimacy and romantic connection creates a strong foundation for a happy and enduring marriage. These efforts require ongoing attention, but they contribute significantly to the long-term success and satisfaction within the relationship.

Intimacy and romance are fundamental principles that contribute to a happy and fulfilling marriage. Intimacy encompasses emotional, physical, and intellectual closeness between partners. It involves sharing thoughts, feelings, and vulnerabilities, which fosters a deep understanding and connection.

Romance adds excitement and passion to a marriage. Thoughtful gestures, surprise dates, and expressions of love keep the spark alive. Regular communication and quality time together help maintain a strong emotional bond.

Physical intimacy is essential too, as it nurtures closeness and releases oxytocin, the "love hormone." Open communication about desires and preferences ensures both partners feel valued and respected.

Sustaining intimacy and romance requires effort from both partners. It involves active listening, empathy, and ongoing communication to adapt to each other's changing needs. Keep in mind that every relationship is unique, so finding what works best for both of you is key to maintaining a happy and fulfilling marriage.

Once upon a time, there was a couple named Sarah and John. They had been married for many years and had faced their fair share of challenges. However, their marriage remained strong and fulfilling because they prioritized intimacy and romance.

Every week, without fail, Sarah and John had a "date night." This was a sacred time for them to connect on a deeper level. They would take turns planning these special evenings, which ranged from candlelit dinners at home to adventurous outings. During these date nights, they put away their phones, focused on each other, and discussed their dreams, fears, and aspirations. They made an effort to truly listen and support one another.

But it wasn't just about the grand gestures. Sarah and John also knew the importance of small, everyday acts of affection. They exchanged sweet notes, surprise gifts, and affectionate gestures regularly. Even after many years of marriage, they continued to hold hands, cuddle on the couch, and say "I love you" every day.

Their friends often admired their relationship, and some even asked for advice. Sarah and John would tell them, "The key is to keep the flame of romance alive. It's not about avoiding conflicts but about navigating them together with love and respect. Intimacy isn't something that just happens; it's something you cultivate."

Through the ups and downs of life, Sarah and John's marriage remained strong, filled with love and passion. They understood that fostering intimacy and romance wasn't just a goal but an ongoing journey, and it was this commitment that made their marriage a truly happy one.

In this story, Sarah and John's commitment to fostering intimacy and romance in their marriage showcases how it can lead to a lasting and fulfilling partnership, serving as a valuable principle for a happy marriage.

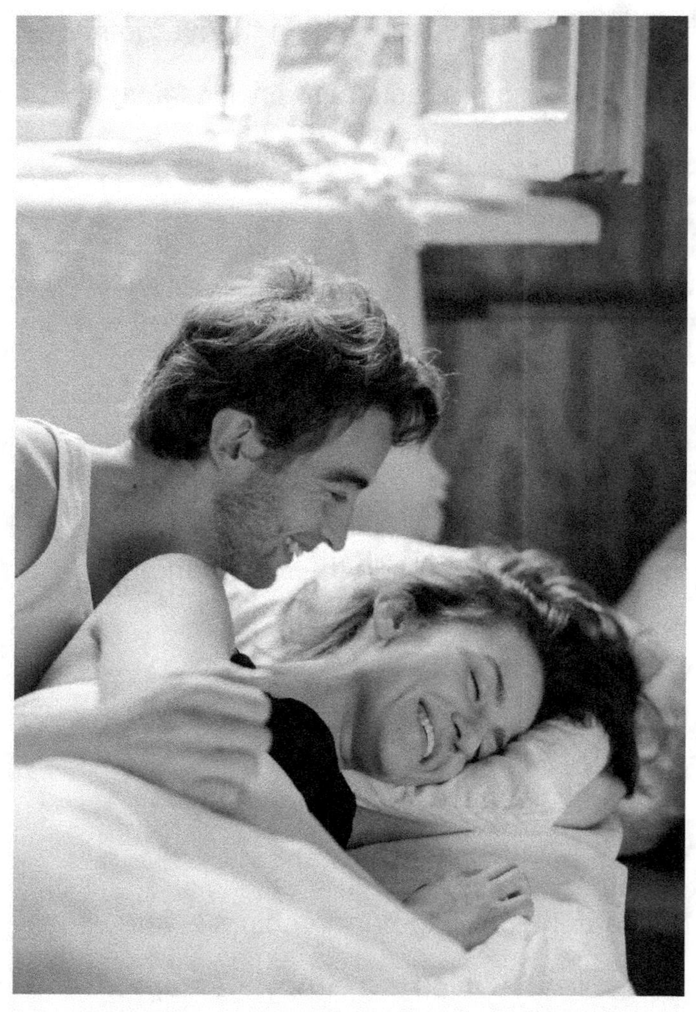

Chapter 6

Resolving Conflict with Grace

Conflicts are a natural part of any relationship. This chapter offers strategies for resolving disagreements with respect and understanding. By cultivating effective conflict resolution skills, couples can transform challenges into opportunities for growth and connection.

"Resolving Conflict with Grace" is a foundational principle for maintaining a happy and healthy marriage. It involves addressing disagreements and differences in a respectful, empathetic, and constructive manner. Here's a more comprehensive overview of how this principle contributes to a successful partnership:

Open Communication: Effective communication is key. Both partners should feel comfortable expressing their thoughts and emotions without fear of judgment. Active listening is equally important, allowing each person to truly understand the other's perspective.

Mutual Respect: Treating each other with respect, even during disagreements, sets the tone for a harmonious relationship. Avoiding belittling comments, sarcasm, or insults is crucial. Focus on the issue at hand instead of attacking your partner's character.

Empathy: Put yourself in your partner's shoes to better understand their feelings and viewpoints. Empathy fosters understanding and can defuse potential conflicts by showing that you value your partner's emotions.

Patience: Conflict resolution takes time. Be patient and allow each other space to process emotions and thoughts. Avoid pushing for immediate solutions, as this can escalate tensions.

Pick the Right Time and Place: Choose an appropriate time and a private, comfortable setting to discuss issues. Avoid confronting problems during high-stress moments or in front of others.

Focus on the Issue, Not the Person: When discussing conflicts, concentrate on the specific problem rather than making it personal. Use "I" statements to express your feelings without blaming or accusing your partner.

Collaborative Problem-Solving: Approach conflicts as a team working toward a solution, rather than competing against each other. Brainstorm possible solutions together and compromise when necessary.

Apologize and Forgive: Apologizing when you're wrong and forgiving when your partner apologizes are crucial steps. Forgiveness doesn't mean forgetting, but it actually means moving forward without holding onto resentment.

Use Humor Wisely: Humor can lighten the mood and help ease tensions, but be cautious not to use sarcasm or jokes that may hurt your partner's feelings.

Seek Professional Help if Needed: There's no shame in seeking counseling or therapy if conflicts become overwhelming or persistent. A neutral third party can provide guidance and tools for effective conflict resolution.

Maintain Perspective: Remember the bigger picture and the reasons you love each other. Sometimes, conflicts are small in the grand scheme of a relationship.

Learn from Each Conflict: Every conflict is an opportunity for you to grow and learn.

Reflect on what you can improve individually and as a couple to prevent same issues in the future.
"Resolving Conflict with Grace" requires ongoing effort, self-awareness, and a genuine commitment to the well-being of the relationship. By following these principles, couples can navigate challenges in a way that strengthens their bond rather than weakening it.

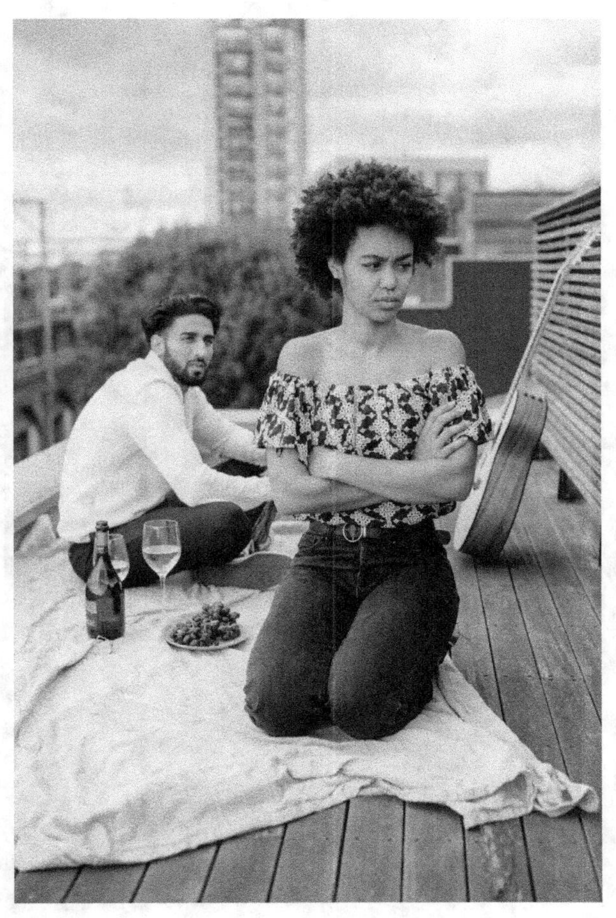

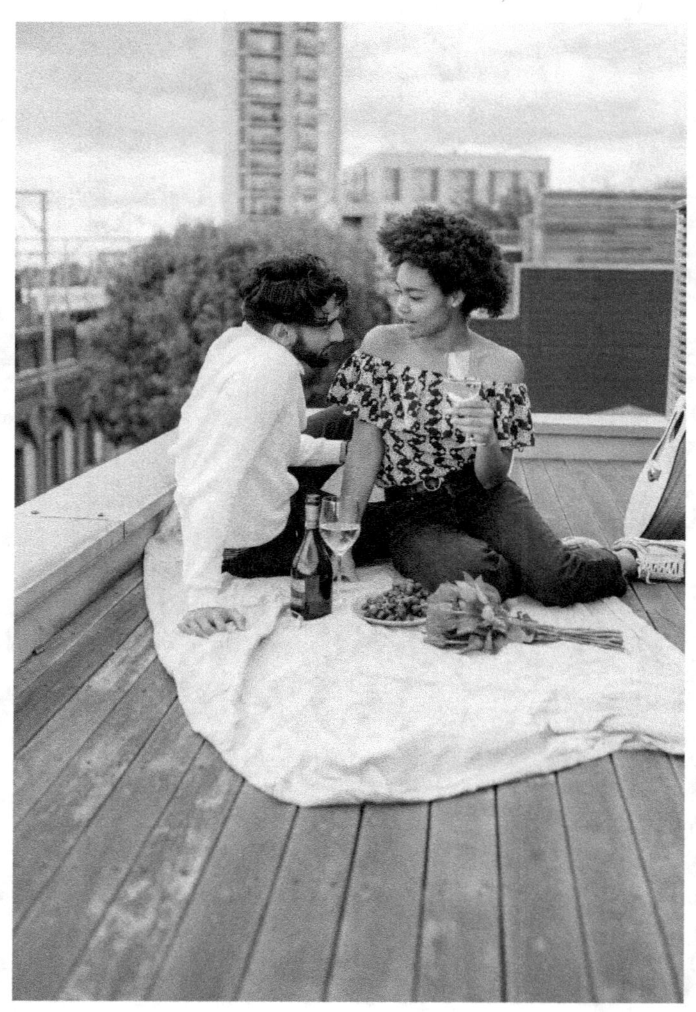

Chapter 7

Forgiveness and Compromise

These two aspects contribute significantly to the longevity and strength of a marital relationship. Let's delve into each concept in more detail:

Forgiveness:

Forgiveness is the act of letting go of resentment, anger, and negative emotions after a hurtful incident. In a marriage, conflicts and misunderstandings are inevitable due to differences in personalities, perspectives, and expectations. However, holding onto grudges can create a toxic environment, eroding trust and emotional intimacy.

Practicing forgiveness in a marriage doesn't mean condoning or excusing hurtful behavior. Instead, it's a conscious decision to release the emotional burden and work towards healing. It requires empathy, understanding, and a willingness to move forward. By forgiving your partner, you not only free them from past mistakes but also liberate yourself from the emotional weight that can hinder the growth of the relationship.

Forgiveness is a fundamental principle of a happy marriage because it allows couples to navigate the inevitable challenges, conflicts, and mistakes that arise in any relationship. Holding onto grudges or refusing to forgive can create a toxic environment of resentment, bitterness, and emotional distance.

Forgiveness promotes open communication and vulnerability, essential components of a strong marriage. It encourages couples to address their issues instead of burying them, leading to greater understanding and growth. When one partner forgives the other, it shows a willingness to let go of past wrongs and work towards a harmonious future.

Additionally, forgiveness fosters empathy and compassion. Recognizing that both partners are fallible and make mistakes helps create an atmosphere of acceptance. It also prevents a "blame game" mentality, encouraging both individuals to take responsibility for their actions and contribute to the relationship's overall well-being.

Ultimately, forgiveness allows a couple to move forward together. It's a way to heal wounds, rebuild trust, and strengthen the emotional bond. Without forgiveness, unresolved conflicts can build up over time, eroding the foundation of the marriage and leading to unhappiness and dissatisfaction.

Remember that forgiveness doesn't mean ignoring serious issues or allowing unhealthy behavior. It's about finding a balance between addressing problems and offering a chance for growth and reconciliation.

Compromise

Compromise involves finding middle ground and making concessions to reach mutual agreements. In a marriage, compromise is essential because each individual brings their own values, preferences, and needs to the relationship. It's unrealistic to expect that two people will always share the same viewpoints or desires.

Compromise in marriage is a vital principle for fostering a happy and lasting relationship. It's about finding middle ground, understanding each other's perspectives, and working together to make joint decisions. Let me share a story to illustrate this point:

Once upon a time, there was a couple named Sarah and Alex. They were deeply in love and decided to get married. Early on, their marriage was filled with joy and excitement, but as time passed, they began to realize their differences.

Sarah was an early riser who valued routine and structure, while Alex was a night owl who preferred spontaneity and flexibility.

Initially, their differences didn't cause major issues, but over time, these contrasting habits led to misunderstandings and conflicts. Sarah felt frustrated because she wanted to spend quality time with Alex in the mornings, while Alex felt stifled by the routine that Sarah insisted upon. Both felt their individual needs weren't being met, and tension began to build.

Recognizing the importance of compromise, they decided to have an open and honest conversation. They shared their feelings, concerns, and desires with each other. Through this dialogue, they realized that their differences weren't problems to solve, but

rather opportunities to learn and grow together.
They decided to compromise by setting some
guidelines for their daily routines that allowed
them to spend quality time together while also
accommodating their personal preferences.

Sarah agreed to occasionally stay up late with
Alex, while Alex committed to waking up earlier
a few times a week. This compromise allowed
them to share moments that were important to
both of them and still maintain their individual
identities. They realized that their marriage
wasn't about erasing differences, but about
finding ways to honor each other's needs.

As the years went by, Sarah and Alex
continued to apply the principle of compromise
in various aspects of their marriage. They
learned that by understanding and respecting

each other's perspectives, they could find solutions that benefited both of them. Their marriage flourished because they embraced compromise as a way to navigate challenges and strengthen their bond.

This story highlights that compromise is a cornerstone of a successful marriage. It's not about one person always giving in, but about both partners making adjustments to accommodate each other's needs and preferences. Through compromise, couples can build trust, empathy, and a deep sense of partnership, laying the foundation for a happy and enduring marriage.

Healthy compromise requires effective communication and a genuine desire to prioritize the well-being of the relationship. It's about finding solutions that satisfy both partners to some extent, even if it means making adjustments and sacrifices. The art of compromise strengthens the bond by demonstrating a willingness to accommodate each other's needs and desires, fostering a sense of teamwork and unity.

Backed by Psychological Insights:

Psychological research supports the significance of forgiveness and compromise in maintaining marital satisfaction. Studies have shown that practicing forgiveness can lead to reduced stress, improved mental health, and increased relationship satisfaction. It contributes to emotional resilience and creates a positive atmosphere that encourages growth and development.

Similarly, compromise has been found to foster better communication skills, reduce conflicts, and enhance relationship stability. Couples who engage in healthy compromise report higher levels of relationship satisfaction and intimacy. This is because compromise nurtures a sense of fairness and equality, promoting a sense of partnership where both individuals feel valued and understood. Accept that conflicts are natural and practice forgiveness. Compromise when needed to find solutions that work for both of you. Certainly, forgiveness and compromise are indeed foundational principles in maintaining a happy and successful marriage.

In conclusion, **forgiveness** and **compromise** serve as cornerstones of a happy marriage. They enable couples to navigate challenges, disagreements, and differences while fostering a strong emotional connection. These principles are rooted in empathy, communication, and a shared commitment to the well-being of the relationship. By practicing forgiveness and compromise, couples can create a nurturing and enduring marital bond that stands the test of time.

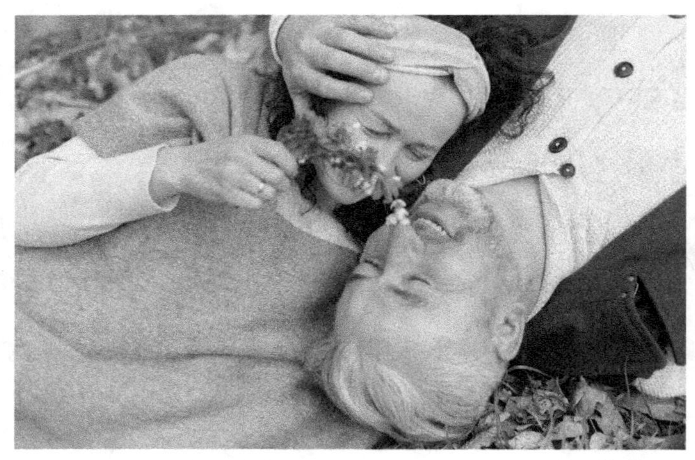

Chapter 8

Prioritizing Self-Care and Individuality

Maintaining a happy marriage involves tending to one's own well-being. This chapter discusses the importance of self-care and individual pursuits within a partnership. When both partners nurture their personal passions, they bring fresh energy and positivity to the marriage.

Prioritizing self-care and individuality within a marriage is crucial for maintaining a healthy and fulfilling relationship. While the idea of focusing on oneself might seem counterintuitive to a partnership, it's actually a key element in ensuring both partners remain content and capable of contributing positively to the relationship.

1. **Personal Growth:** Encouraging individuality allows each partner to continue growing as a person. Pursuing hobbies, interests, and personal goals can lead to self-discovery and personal development. When both individuals are thriving personally, it can bring more vibrancy and enthusiasm to the marriage.

2. **Preventing Resentment:** Neglecting one's own needs for the sake of the relationship can lead to resentment over time. Prioritizing self-care ensures that each partner's emotional and physical needs are met, reducing the likelihood

of harboring negative feelings towards the other person.

3. **Maintaining Identity:** A strong sense of self is fundamental to maintaining one's identity within a marriage. It's important to remember that while you're a part of a couple, you're also an individual with unique desires and aspirations. Valuing your own identity can prevent feelings of being consumed by the relationship.

4. **Healthy Communication:** Pursuing self-care fosters open communication about each partner's needs and boundaries. Discussing personal goals and how to support each other in achieving them leads to a deeper understanding of one another, enhancing overall communication in the relationship.

5. **Reducing Dependency:** Relying solely on your partner for happiness can put unnecessary strain on the relationship. When both individuals actively engage in self-care, they become less dependent on each other for emotional fulfillment, which can lead to a more balanced and sustainable partnership.

6. **Quality Time:** Prioritizing individuality doesn't mean neglecting the relationship. It can actually enhance the quality of the time spent together. When partners have their own interests and experiences to share, conversations become richer and more engaging.

7. **Respecting Boundaries:** Respecting each other's need for personal space and time can prevent feelings of suffocation. It allows for moments of

solitude, which can be rejuvenating and necessary for mental well-being.

8. **Role Modeling:** Demonstrating self-care and individuality sets a positive example for any children in the family. It teaches them that healthy relationships involve respecting each other's autonomy and fostering personal growth.

9. **Longevity:** Couples who prioritize self-care and individuality often report higher levels of marital satisfaction and longevity. When partners are content in their own lives, they bring positivity and a sense of fulfillment to the relationship, enhancing overall happiness.

Remember that **balance** is key. While individuality and self-care are essential, it's also important to find ways to connect and share experiences as a couple. Building a strong foundation of personal well-being within the context of a partnership can lead to a lasting and fulfilling marriage.

Chapter 9

Embracing Laughter and Playfulness

Laughter is the glue that binds hearts together. This chapter explores the value of injecting humor and playfulness into daily life. Through shared laughter, couples create joyful memories that reinforce their bond.

Embracing laughter and playfulness as a principle of a happy marriage involves infusing a sense of joy, humor, and light-heartedness into the relationship. It means finding opportunities to laugh together, share jokes, and engage in playful activities that create a positive and relaxed atmosphere. This principle has several benefits:

1. **Stress Relief:** Life's challenges can be easier to handle when couples can find humor in tough situations. Playful moments can serve as a temporary escape from stress, allowing both partners to reset and face difficulties with a clearer perspective.

2. **Bond Strengthening:** Sharing laughter creates a unique bond. Inside jokes and playful memories become cherished aspects of the relationship, fostering a sense of intimacy and connection that strengthens over time.

3. **Communication:** Playfulness encourages open communication and non-verbal cues. Couples often use playful banter and gestures to express affection and resolve conflicts, making it

easier to address sensitive topics
without excessive tension.

4. **Resilience:** Couples who can laugh
    together tend to be more resilient in the
    face of challenges. Playfulness
    promotes adaptability, enabling partners
    to navigate changes and uncertainties
    while maintaining a positive outlook.

5. **Rediscovering Fun:** Over time,
    responsibilities and routines can make a
    relationship feel monotonous.
    Embracing playfulness helps couples
    rediscover the fun and excitement that
    initially drew them together, reigniting
    the spark.

6. **Positive Environment:** A marriage
    filled with laughter and playfulness
    creates a positive home environment
    that benefits not only the couple but also

any children or family members involved. It sets a tone of joy and optimism that permeates daily interactions.

7. **Fostering Creativity:** Playfulness encourages creativity and innovation, both individually and as a couple. Trying new activities, exploring hobbies, and engaging in imaginative play can lead to personal growth and shared experiences.

8. **Celebrating Togetherness:** Playful moments provide opportunities to celebrate each other's company. Whether through game nights, playful outings, or simple shared jokes, couples can find joy in just being around one another.

To implement this principle, couples can **schedule** regular moments of playfulness, engage in activities that make them both laugh, create a safe space for lighthearted teasing, and be open to finding humor in everyday situations. It's important to remember that while embracing laughter and playfulness, maintaining respect and sensitivity to each other's boundaries is key.

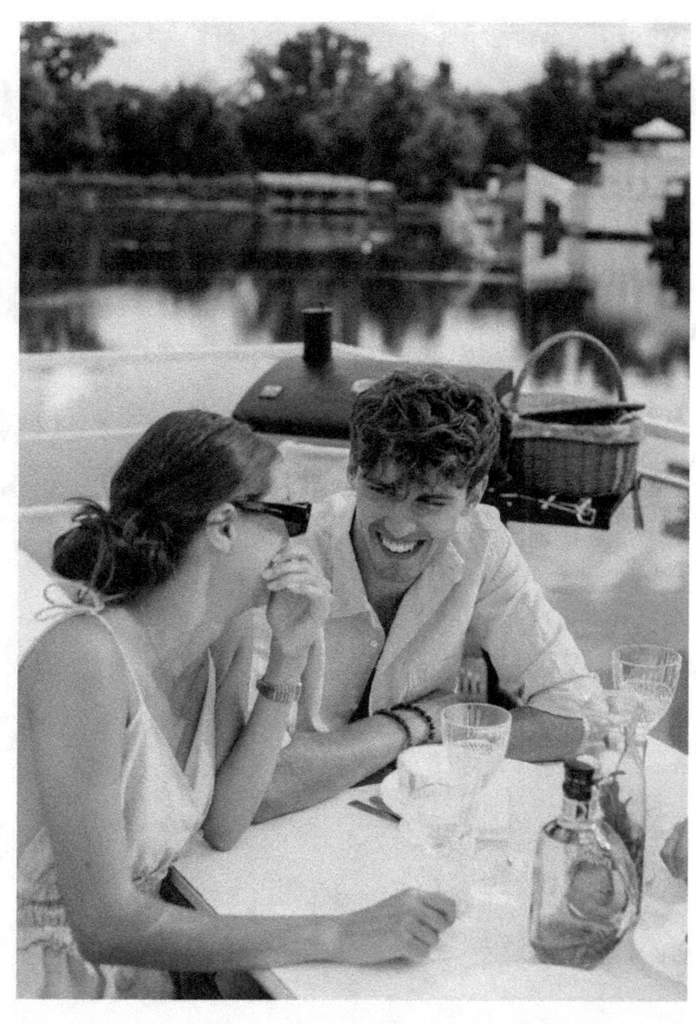

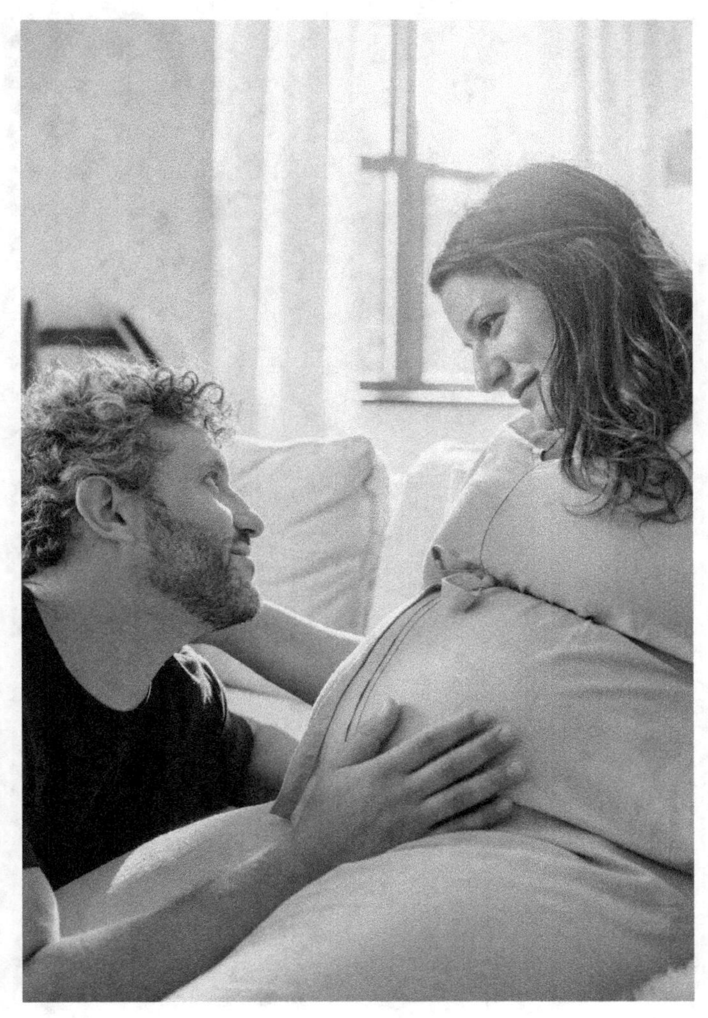

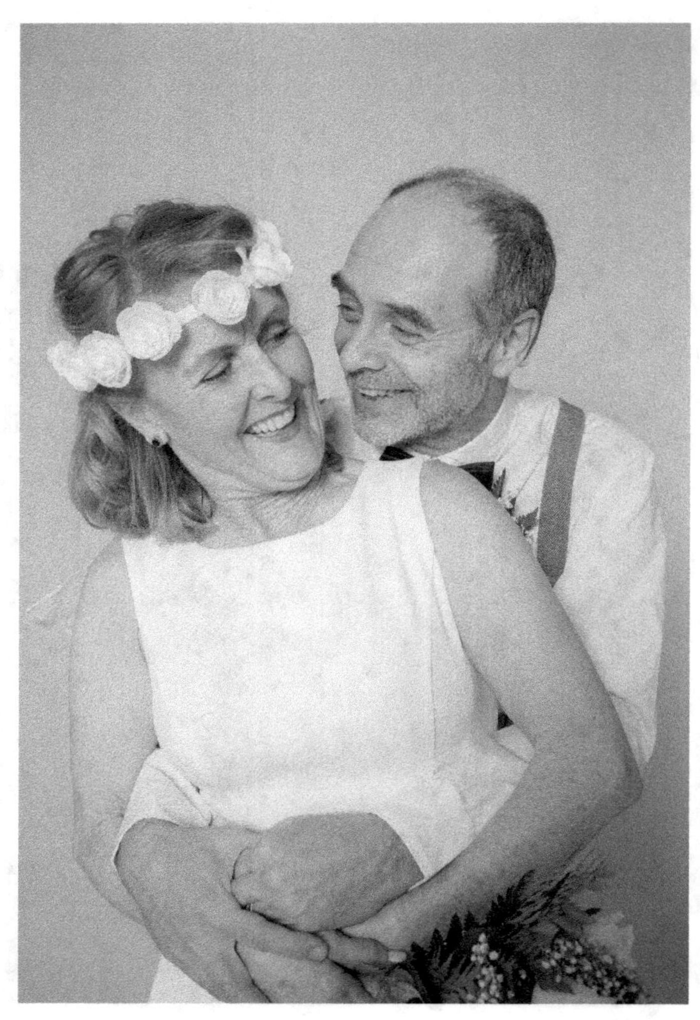

Chapter 10

Sustaining Marriage Commitment

"Sustaining Commitment through Time" is indeed a crucial principle for a happy marriage. It involves continuously nurturing the emotional connection, communication, and understanding between partners as the years go by. This includes showing appreciation, adapting to changes, and being patient during challenging times. Regularly reinforcing your commitment can help maintain a strong and fulfilling marital bond.

Open communication, mutual respect, shared goals, and adapting to changes together are key principles to maintain that commitment. Regularly investing time and effort into your relationship, showing appreciation, and finding ways to keep the romance alive can help strengthen the bond and lead to a fulfilling and lasting

Sustaining a marriage commitment brings several benefits to a happy marriage. It fosters trust, emotional intimacy, and stability, providing a strong foundation for both partners. Commitment helps navigate challenges, as both individuals are more likely to work through difficulties rather than giving up. Over time, commitment can lead to deeper understanding and appreciation of each other, enhancing the overall quality of the relationship.

Sustaining marriage commitment is indeed a fundamental principle for a happy and enduring marriage. Here's an elaboration on why it's crucial:

Foundation of Trust: Commitment forms the foundation of trust in a marriage. When both partners are committed to the relationship, they feel secure and can rely on each other emotionally, which is essential for a happy marriage.

Weathering Challenges: Every marriage faces challenges, be it financial difficulties, conflicts, or external stressors. Commitment means you're both willing to work through these challenges together, rather than giving up when times get tough.

Long-Term Perspective: A committed couple focuses on the long-term perspective of their marriage. They understand that there will be ups and downs but are determined to grow old together. This perspective helps in making compromises and sacrifices for the greater good of the relationship.

Emotional Connection: Commitment fosters a deeper emotional connection. Knowing that your partner is there for you through thick and thin creates a sense of intimacy and bonding that contributes to marital happiness.

Conflict Resolution: Commitment encourages healthy conflict resolution. Instead of resorting to destructive arguments or seeking separation, committed partners are more likely to seek compromise, communicate openly, and find solutions that strengthen their relationship.

Family Stability: For couples with children, commitment is vital for providing a stable family environment. Children benefit greatly from the security of knowing their parents are committed to each other and the family unit.

Personal Growth: Commitment can also support personal growth. In a committed relationship, individuals often find support and encouragement to become the best versions of themselves.

Shared Goals: Committed couples tend to have shared goals and dreams, which can give their marriage a sense of purpose and direction. Pursuing these goals together can be fulfilling and contribute to happiness.

Respect and Love: Commitment is a manifestation of respect and love for your partner. It's a daily choice to prioritize their happiness and well-being, which in turn fosters mutual respect and love.

Model for Others: A committed marriage can serve as a positive model for friends and family. It demonstrates the value of working through challenges and staying devoted to one another, potentially influencing others in a positive way.

In summary, sustaining marriage commitment involves continuously choosing to prioritize and invest in your relationship. It's the glue that holds a marriage together during both the good and challenging times, ultimately leading to a happier and more fulfilling relationship.

Chapter 11

Faithfulness

Faithfulness, as a fundamental principle of a thriving marriage, is rooted in trust, respect, and emotional security. It encompasses unwavering loyalty, honesty, and the commitment to remaining exclusive to one's partner. This principle involves both physical and emotional fidelity, ensuring that the bond between spouses remains strong and unbreakable.

In a marriage built on faithfulness, couples find solace in knowing that they can rely on each other through life's challenges. The absence of doubt about a partner's intentions fosters an environment of openness and effective communication, as both individuals feel comfortable sharing their thoughts and feelings without fear of betrayal. This contributes to a deeper emotional connection and helps resolve conflicts in a healthy manner.

Faithfulness acts as a shield against external temptations, as individuals prioritize the sanctity of their marital commitment over fleeting desires. By resisting the allure of infidelity, couples maintain a sense of integrity and honor, bolstering the love and admiration they hold for one another. This dedication not only enhances the bond between partners but also serves as a positive example for any children in the family, teaching them the values of respect, commitment, and responsibility.

Moreover, faithfulness contributes to the development of a strong sense of identity as a couple. Knowing that their partner is devoted exclusively to them, individuals can fully invest in the relationship without fear of abandonment or betrayal. This foundation of trust enables both partners to grow personally and together, as they support each other's dreams, aspirations, and personal growth.

Incorporating faithfulness into a marriage requires ongoing effort. Regular expressions of love, appreciation, and affirmation help fortify the emotional connection, reducing the likelihood of seeking validation elsewhere. Couples can also engage in activities that strengthen their bond, such as quality time spent together, shared interests, and ongoing emotional intimacy.

Once upon a time, in a quaint village nestled between rolling hills, lived a couple named Lillian and Samuel. Their love story was a testament to the principle of faithfulness in a happy marriage. From the day they met at the village fair, their connection was palpable, like a melody that resonates in the heart.

Lillian was an artist, her vibrant spirit mirroring the vivid colors she painted onto canvas. Samuel, on the other hand, was a skilled carpenter, crafting intricate pieces that showcased his dedication to his work. Their differences only seemed to deepen their bond, as they embraced each other's passions and supported their dreams.

Through life's highs and lows, Lillian and Samuel remained unwaveringly faithful to each other. When the stormy winds of doubt threatened to creep in, they stood strong, rooted in the foundation of trust they had built over the years. Their love was like a majestic oak tree, growing steadily with time, its branches spreading wide to shelter them from life's challenges.

One summer, Samuel fell gravely ill, and the village was abuzz with concern. Lillian stood by his side, nursing him back to health with a tenderness that spoke volumes of her devotion. Even in his weakest moments, Samuel would gaze at her with eyes full of gratitude, knowing that his life was intertwined with someone who would stand by him through any storm.

As years turned into decades, their love story remained an inspiration to all who knew them. Their children grew up witnessing a partnership built on unwavering loyalty and support, a love story that was not without its flaws but was always marked by a commitment to work through challenges together.

Lillian and Samuel's story reminds us that faithfulness is not just about staying faithful physically, but also emotionally and spiritually. It's about being there for each other through the mundane and the extraordinary, through joy and sorrow, through dreams achieved and those yet to be realized.

Their love story echoes through time, a living testament to the beauty of faithfulness in a happy marriage, a reminder that true love is a

tapestry woven with threads of trust,
commitment, and a shared journey that only
grows more beautiful with each passing day.

In essence, faithfulness serves as a
cornerstone of a happy marriage, fostering an
environment of trust, commitment, and
emotional security. By upholding this principle,
couples ensure the longevity of their
relationship, creating a foundation upon which
they can build a life of shared happiness,
growth, and fulfillment.

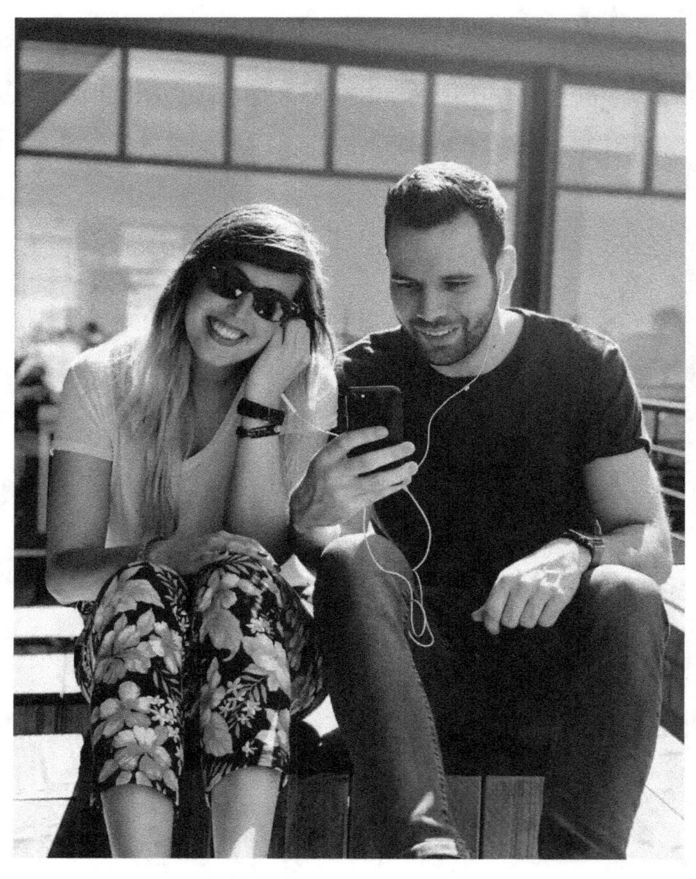

Chapter 12

LOVE

Love is often considered the cornerstone of a happy and fulfilling marriage. It's the powerful force that binds two individuals together, providing the emotional sustenance needed to weather life's storms and celebrate its joys. But love in marriage is not a simplistic or one-dimensional concept; it encompasses a multitude of dimensions that contribute to a harmonious and lasting partnership. Love is the glue that holds a marriage together through thick and thin.

Certainly, love is a fundamental principle in a happy marriage, and here are some additional passages that emphasize its importance:

First and foremost, love in a marriage is characterized by emotional intimacy. This means not only sharing your feelings but also being a supportive and empathetic listener. In a loving marriage, couples create a safe space where they can openly express their thoughts,

concerns, and vulnerabilities. This emotional connection builds trust and a sense of security, allowing both partners to be themselves without fear of judgment.
Love creates a deep emotional and physical connection. It's about intimacy that goes beyond the physical realm and includes emotional vulnerability. This connection keeps the spark alive in a marriage.

Another critical aspect of love in marriage is respect. Love goes hand in hand with admiration and appreciation for your partner. It involves recognizing and valuing their unique qualities, ideas, and perspectives. Respect means treating your spouse as an equal, honoring their boundaries, and actively showing appreciation for their contributions to the relationship.

Communication is the lifeblood of any successful marriage, and love is expressed through effective and open communication. Honest and respectful dialogue fosters understanding and helps resolve conflicts. Loving couples prioritize clear and transparent communication, which prevents misunderstandings and nurtures a sense of unity. Love thrives on open and honest communication. It means sharing your thoughts, fears, and aspirations with your partner. Love is the driving force behind the desire to connect through words.

Forgiveness and compassion are essential components of love within a marriage. No one is perfect, and conflicts are inevitable. Love allows couples to navigate these challenges with grace and understanding. Forgiving one another's mistakes and showing compassion during difficult times are demonstrations of love's enduring power.
 Love allows for forgiveness and growth. Inevitably, mistakes happen, but love means forgiving and learning together. It's about recognizing that nobody is perfect and that a strong marriage is built on forgiveness and the willingness to move forward.

Love in marriage also thrives on shared experiences and quality time together. Building a life together involves creating cherished memories, pursuing common interests, and supporting each other's dreams and aspirations. These shared moments reinforce the bond between spouses and serve as a reminder of the love that brought them together. Love binds two people together in pursuit of common dreams and goals. It's the driving force that makes partners want to build a life together, create a family, and face the future hand in hand.

Love encourages personal and joint growth. It's about supporting each other's individual journeys and growing together as a couple. Love is the motivation to become the best versions of yourselves.
 Love brings joy and laughter into a marriage. It's about finding joy in the simple moments and sharing laughter, even during challenging times. Love adds brightness and positivity to daily life.

 Trust is the foundation upon which love is built. It is earned through consistency, honesty, and reliability. When trust exists within a marriage, it bolsters the sense of security and commitment, allowing love to flourish.
 Love is built on mutual respect and trust. In a happy marriage, partners trust each other

implicitly, knowing that they have each other's best interests at heart. Love is the foundation upon which this trust is established and maintained.

Love fosters empathy and understanding. It means taking the time to truly listen and understand your partner's feelings, even when they're difficult to express. It's about putting yourself in their shoes and showing compassion.

Love in a marriage means being each other's biggest cheerleaders. It's about providing unwavering support through life's ups and downs. When you love your partner deeply, you stand by them, no matter what.

In a happy marriage, love is not just a fleeting emotion; it's a guiding principle that underlies every aspect of the relationship, creating a strong and enduring bond between two people. Lastly, love in marriage evolves over time. It's not static but rather a dynamic force that adapts to the changing circumstances of life. It deepens and matures as couples face life's challenges together and continue to invest in their relationship.

In conclusion, love is the guiding principle of a happy marriage, encompassing emotional intimacy, respect, communication, forgiveness, compassion, shared experiences, trust, and evolution. When nurtured and cherished, love creates a strong and enduring foundation for a lifelong journey of love and partnership.

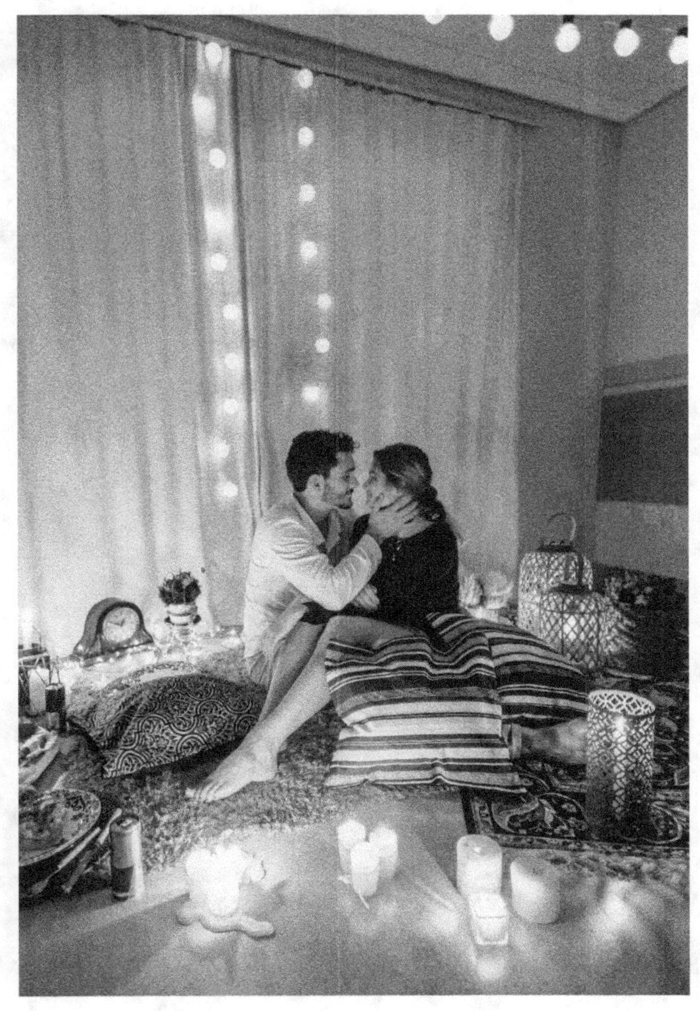

Conclusion

- **"Happy Marriage"** encapsulates the essence of a joyful and everlasting marriage through its exploration of open communication, trust, growth, shared values, intimacy, conflict resolution, self-care, playfulness, and unwavering commitment. By embracing these principles, couples can embark on a journey of love, understanding, and shared happiness that stands the test of time.

- In the journey towards a fulfilling and enduring marital bond, the principles outlined in this book serve as guiding lights. A happy marriage is not a destination but a continuous exploration of each other's worlds, fueled by love, understanding, and shared experiences. As we conclude our exploration of the principles that underpin a joyous union, let's reflect on the key takeaways that can contribute to a harmonious and lasting partnership.

- **1. Communication**: Open and honest communication forms the cornerstone of a thriving marriage. The ability to express thoughts, feelings, and concerns fosters mutual understanding and prevents misunderstandings from festering.

- **2. Trust and Respect:** Trust is the bedrock upon which a strong marriage is built. By honoring commitments and respecting each other's boundaries, couples create an environment where both feel secure and valued.

- **3. Empathy and Understanding:** Walking in your partner's shoes fosters empathy and strengthens the emotional connection. Understanding each other's perspectives paves the way for compromise and solutions during challenging times.

- **4. Shared Goals:** Setting common goals, whether they relate to career, family, or personal growth, provides a sense of purpose and direction. Striving towards these goals together enhances cooperation and unity.

- **5. Quality Time:** Spending quality time together strengthens the emotional bond. Whether through shared hobbies, date nights, or simply being present, carving out moments to connect is essential.

- **6. Flexibility and Patience:** The ability to adapt to change and exhibit patience during trying times prevents unnecessary friction. Flexibility allows couples to weather life's storms while deepening their connection.

- **7. Intimacy:** Physical and emotional intimacy are vital components of a happy marriage. Nurturing these aspects ensures that the relationship remains vibrant and satisfying.

- **8. Conflict Resolution:** Disagreements are inevitable, but the way they are resolved can either strengthen or weaken a marriage. Practicing active listening, seeking common ground, and showing appreciation for each other's viewpoints contribute to healthy conflict resolution.

- **9. Appreciation and Affection:**
  Expressing appreciation for each other's
  contributions and showing affection
  through words and gestures reinforces
  the love between partners.

- **10. Continuous Growth:** A happy
  marriage is a journey of personal and
  joint growth. Embracing change,
  learning from experiences, and evolving
  together keeps the relationship dynamic
  and fulfilling.

- **In closing**, a happy marriage isn't
  without its challenges, but armed with
  these principles, couples can navigate
  the highs and lows with grace and
  resilience. Remember that the pursuit of
  happiness in marriage is a daily
  commitment, a promise to stand by
  each other through all seasons of life.

As you embark on this lifelong
adventure, may the wisdom shared in
this book illuminate your path to a
joyous and enduring marriage.

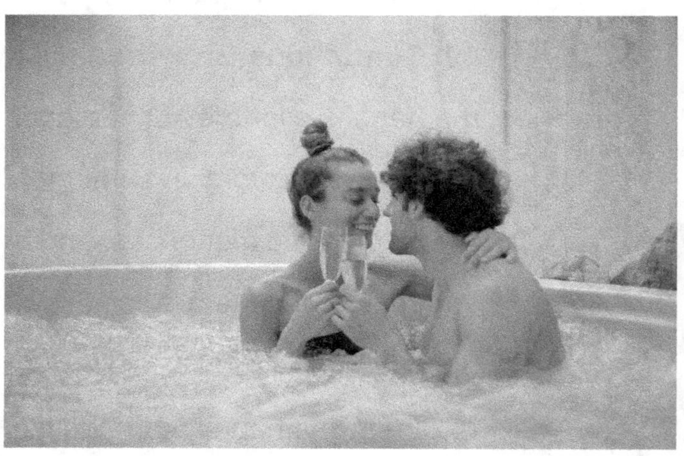

9 798862 174809